Table Of Contents

Chapter 1: Understanding Fitness in Your 40s

The Importance of Fitness in Your 40s

In your 40s, maintaining a healthy level of fitness becomes even more crucial. This is the time in your life when your metabolism starts to slow down, making it easier to gain weight and harder to lose it. But fear not, because with the right mindset and dedication, you can overcome these age-related challenges and stay in shape. By incorporating regular exercise, a balanced diet, and proper nutrition, you can achieve your fitness goals and maintain a strong and healthy body well into your 40s and beyond.

One of the key aspects of staying fit in your 40s is to focus on losing weight and building muscle. As we age, our muscle mass naturally decreases, which can lead to a slower metabolism and weight gain. By incorporating strength training exercises into your workout routine, you can build muscle, increase your metabolism, and burn more calories throughout the day. Combine this with cardiovascular exercises like running, cycling, or swimming to help shed those extra pounds and improve your overall fitness level.

Flexibility and mobility are also important factors to consider in your 40s. As we age, our joints can become stiff and our range of motion can decrease, making it harder to perform everyday activities and exercises. By incorporating stretching exercises and mobility drills into your routine, you can improve your flexibility, reduce the risk of injury, and enhance your overall athletic performance. Yoga, Pilates, and foam rolling are great options to help improve your flexibility and mobility in your 40s.

Maintaining a healthy diet and nutrition plan is essential for overall health and fitness, especially in your 40s. Eating a well-balanced diet rich in fruits, vegetables, lean proteins, and whole grains can help fuel your workouts, boost your metabolism, and support muscle recovery and growth. Avoiding processed foods, sugary drinks, and excessive amounts of alcohol can also help you maintain a healthy weight and reduce the risk of developing chronic diseases. Remember, food is fuel for your body, so choose wisely and nourish yourself with nutrient-dense foods to support your fitness goals.

In your 40s, it's important to listen to your body and adjust your fitness routine accordingly. Be mindful of any age-related fitness challenges you may face, such as joint pain, arthritis, or decreased energy levels. If you experience any discomfort or pain, consult with a healthcare professional or a fitness trainer to modify your workouts and prevent injuries. By staying active, setting realistic fitness goals, and staying consistent with your routine, you can overcome these challenges and maintain a healthy and active lifestyle in your 40s. Remember, it's never too late to start prioritizing your health and fitness, so embrace this new chapter in your life with determination and enthusiasm.

Common Fitness Challenges in Your 40s

As we enter our 40s, we may find ourselves facing new challenges when it comes to our fitness journey. It's important to acknowledge that our bodies may not respond to exercise and diet in the same way they did in our younger years. However, with the right mindset and approach, we can overcome these challenges and continue to lead a healthy and active lifestyle.

One common challenge that many individuals face in their 40s is the difficulty of losing weight and building muscle. Our metabolism tends to slow down as we age, making it more challenging to shed those extra pounds and maintain muscle mass. However, with a combination of strength training, cardiovascular exercise, and a balanced diet, it is still possible to achieve your fitness goals. Remember, consistency is key, and progress may be slower than before, but every small step counts towards your ultimate success.

Another challenge that often arises in our 40s is a decrease in flexibility and mobility. Years of sitting at a desk or engaging in repetitive movements can lead to tight muscles and limited range of motion. Incorporating stretching exercises, yoga, and mobility drills into your routine can help improve flexibility and prevent injuries. Don't be discouraged if you're not as flexible as you once were - with dedication and patience, you can regain your mobility and move with ease.

Maintaining a healthy diet and nutrition plan becomes increasingly important as we age. Our bodies require different nutrients to support optimal health and function, and it's essential to fuel ourselves with whole foods that provide the necessary vitamins and minerals. Planning your meals ahead of time, staying hydrated, and avoiding processed foods can help you stay on track with your nutrition goals. Remember, it's never too late to start making healthier choices and nourishing your body from the inside out.

Lastly, it's crucial to listen to your body and make adjustments as needed to prevent and manage injuries while staying active in your 40s. Pay attention to any aches or pains, and don't push yourself beyond your limits. Incorporate rest days into your routine, prioritize proper form and technique, and consult with a healthcare professional if you experience any persistent discomfort. By taking care of your body and being mindful of your limitations, you can continue to stay active and enjoy the benefits of a consistent fitness routine well into your 40s and beyond. Remember, it's never too late to prioritize your health and well-being - you have the power to make positive changes and lead a balanced and fulfilling life at any age.

Setting Realistic Fitness Goals

Setting realistic fitness goals is crucial for anyone over 40 who wants to improve their health and well-being. As we age, our bodies may not respond to exercise and diet the same way they did in our younger years. However, this doesn't mean that achieving your fitness goals is impossible - it just means that you may need to approach them in a different way.

When setting fitness goals in your 40s, it's important to be realistic about what you can achieve. While it's great to aim high and challenge yourself, setting goals that are too ambitious can lead to frustration and disappointment. Instead, focus on setting small, achievable goals that will help you make steady progress towards your ultimate fitness objectives.

One way to ensure that your fitness goals are realistic is to consult with a fitness professional or trainer who can help you create a personalized plan based on your age, fitness level, and any existing health conditions. They can also provide guidance on how to safely increase the intensity of your workouts and adjust your diet to support your fitness goals.

Another key aspect of setting realistic fitness goals in your 40s is to take into consideration your work, family, and other commitments. Balancing these responsibilities can be challenging, but with proper planning and time management, you can find ways to incorporate exercise and healthy eating into your daily routine. Remember, taking care of yourself is not selfish - it's essential for your overall well-being and ability to fulfill your other obligations.

By setting realistic fitness goals in your 40s, you can improve your physical health, boost your energy levels, and enhance your overall quality of life. Remember to celebrate your progress, no matter how small, and stay motivated by focusing on the positive changes you are making in your body and mind. With dedication and perseverance, you can achieve your fitness goals and enjoy a healthier, more active lifestyle well into your 40s and beyond.

Chapter 2: Overcoming Age-Related Fitness Challenges

Dealing with Slower Metabolism

Dealing with a slower metabolism can be a common challenge for many of us as we enter our 40s. It's important to remember that it's a natural part of the aging process, but there are definitely ways to combat it and keep your metabolism running efficiently. One key strategy is to focus on building muscle through strength training exercises. Muscle mass naturally decreases as we age, so by incorporating weight-bearing exercises into your routine, you can help boost your metabolism and burn more calories even at rest.

In addition to strength training, incorporating high-intensity interval training (HIIT) into your workouts can also help rev up your metabolism. HIIT workouts involve short bursts of intense exercise followed by brief periods of rest, and studies have shown that they can be highly effective at increasing metabolic rate. Plus, they're a great way to fit in a quick and efficient workout, perfect for those with busy schedules.

Another important aspect of dealing with a slower metabolism is ensuring you're getting enough quality sleep. Lack of sleep can disrupt your body's hormone levels, including those that regulate metabolism, so aim for 7-9 hours of restful sleep each night. Additionally, staying hydrated and eating a balanced diet rich in lean proteins, fruits, vegetables, and whole grains can also help keep your metabolism running smoothly.

It's also important to listen to your body and give it the rest and recovery it needs. As we age, our bodies may require more time to recover from workouts, so don't push yourself too hard and make sure to incorporate rest days into your routine. This will help prevent burnout and reduce the risk of injury, allowing you to stay consistent with your fitness goals in the long run.

Remember, everyone's metabolism is different, and it's important to find what works best for you. By incorporating these strategies into your routine and staying consistent with your fitness goals, you can overcome age-related challenges and maintain a healthy metabolism well into your 40s and beyond. Stay positive, stay motivated, and remember that it's never too late to prioritize your health and well-being.

Managing Joint Pain and Stiffness

Managing joint pain and stiffness can be a common challenge as we age, but there are strategies you can implement to alleviate discomfort and improve your overall mobility. One key aspect is to prioritize exercises that focus on flexibility and range of motion, such as yoga or tai chi. These gentle practices can help improve joint function and reduce stiffness over time.

In addition to incorporating flexibility exercises into your routine, it's important to maintain a healthy weight to reduce the strain on your joints. By focusing on a balanced diet and regular exercise, you can not only prevent weight gain but also build muscle to support your joints and improve overall strength. Remember, it's never too late to start making positive changes for your health and well-being.

Another important factor in managing joint pain and stiffness is to listen to your body and give yourself time to rest and recover. Overdoing it with high-impact activities can exacerbate existing issues, so be sure to mix up your routine with low-impact exercises like swimming or cycling. It's all about finding the right balance that works for you and your body.

If you do experience joint pain, don't ignore it. Consult with a healthcare professional or physical therapist to develop a personalized plan that addresses your specific needs and concerns. They can provide guidance on proper form, modifications, and exercises that can help alleviate discomfort and improve your overall joint health.

Remember, managing joint pain and stiffness is a journey, not a race. Be patient with yourself as you work towards improving your mobility and overall well-being. By staying consistent with your exercise routine, maintaining a healthy diet, and seeking professional guidance when needed, you can overcome age-related fitness challenges and continue to lead an active and fulfilling life in your 40s and beyond.

Adapting to Changes in Muscle Mass

Adapting to changes in muscle mass can be a key component of maintaining a healthy and active lifestyle in your 40s. As we age, our bodies naturally lose muscle mass, which can lead to a decrease in strength and metabolism. However, with the right approach, it is possible to build and maintain muscle mass well into your 40s and beyond. By incorporating strength training exercises into your fitness routine, you can help counteract the effects of aging on your muscles and improve your overall health and wellness.

One of the best ways to build muscle after 40 is to focus on compound exercises that target multiple muscle groups at once. Exercises like squats, deadlifts, and bench presses are great for building strength and muscle mass efficiently. Additionally, incorporating resistance training with weights or resistance bands can help stimulate muscle growth and improve muscle tone. By gradually increasing the intensity of your workouts and challenging your muscles with new exercises, you can continue to see improvements in muscle mass and strength over time.

In addition to strength training, it is important to pay attention to your diet and nutrition plan in order to support muscle growth and recovery. Eating a balanced diet that includes plenty of protein, healthy fats, and complex carbohydrates can help fuel your workouts and provide your muscles with the nutrients they need to repair and grow. It is also important to stay hydrated and consume enough calories to support your energy needs and muscle-building goals. By focusing on nutrient-dense foods and staying consistent with your eating habits, you can support your muscle-building efforts and maintain a healthy weight in your 40s.

As you work on building muscle in your 40s, it is important to listen to your body and pay attention to any signs of injury or overtraining. It is normal to experience some muscle soreness and fatigue after intense workouts, but persistent pain or discomfort could be a sign that you need to adjust your routine or seek help from a fitness professional. By practicing proper form, warming up before workouts, and giving your muscles time to rest and recover, you can prevent injuries and stay active and healthy in your 40s.

Ultimately, adapting to changes in muscle mass in your 40s is about finding a balance between challenging yourself and taking care of your body. By incorporating strength training, supporting your muscles with a healthy diet, and listening to your body's needs, you can build and maintain muscle mass as you age. Remember that progress takes time and consistency, so stay patient and stay motivated on your fitness journey. With dedication and perseverance, you can achieve your fitness goals and enjoy a strong and healthy body well into your 40s and beyond.

Chapter 3: Building Muscle and Losing Weight After 40

Strength Training for Muscle Mass

Strength training is a crucial component of any fitness routine, especially for those in their 40s looking to build muscle mass and maintain a healthy weight. By incorporating regular strength training exercises into your workout regimen, you can effectively increase muscle mass, boost your metabolism, and improve overall physical strength. It's never too late to start strength training, and the benefits are well worth the effort.

As we age, our bodies naturally lose muscle mass and strength, making it even more important to prioritize strength training in our fitness routines. By engaging in activities like weightlifting, resistance band exercises, and bodyweight workouts, you can effectively build and maintain muscle mass, which is essential for overall health and functionality. Additionally, strength training can help prevent age-related muscle loss, improve bone density, and enhance overall physical performance.

Incorporating strength training exercises into your workout routine can also help improve flexibility and mobility, which are key components of maintaining a healthy and active lifestyle in your 40s. By focusing on exercises that target different muscle groups and promote joint mobility, you can increase your range of motion, reduce the risk of injury, and enhance your overall flexibility. This can be especially beneficial for those who may be experiencing stiffness or limited mobility due to age-related factors.

When it comes to strength training for muscle mass, it's important to also pay attention to your diet and nutrition plan. Consuming an adequate amount of protein, healthy fats, and carbohydrates is essential for supporting muscle growth and recovery. Additionally, staying hydrated and fueling your body with nutrient-dense foods can help optimize your workouts and promote overall health and well-being. By maintaining a balanced and healthy diet, you can enhance the benefits of your strength training routine and achieve your fitness goals more effectively.

In conclusion, strength training is a powerful tool for anyone over 40 looking to build muscle mass, improve flexibility and mobility, and maintain a healthy weight. By incorporating regular strength training exercises into your fitness routine, you can boost your metabolism, increase muscle mass, and enhance overall physical strength. Remember to focus on proper form, stay consistent with your workouts, and listen to your body's needs. With dedication and perseverance, you can achieve your fitness goals and enjoy the many benefits of strength training well into your 40s and beyond.

Cardiovascular Exercise for Weight Loss

Cardiovascular exercise is a crucial component of any weight loss journey, especially for those of us in our 40s. As we age, our metabolism naturally slows down, making it more challenging to shed those extra pounds. However, incorporating regular cardio workouts into your routine can help rev up your metabolism and burn calories more efficiently. Whether you enjoy running, cycling, swimming, or dancing, find an activity that gets your heart rate up and stick with it to see results.

One of the great things about cardiovascular exercise is that it not only helps with weight loss but also improves your overall cardiovascular health. As we age, our risk for heart disease and other cardiovascular issues increases, so it's important to prioritize activities that keep our hearts strong and healthy. By engaging in regular cardio workouts, you can lower your blood pressure, reduce your risk of heart disease, and improve your overall cardiovascular fitness.

In addition to its physical benefits, cardiovascular exercise can also have a positive impact on your mental health. Physical activity releases endorphins, which are your body's natural mood lifters. This can help combat feelings of stress, anxiety, and depression that often come with juggling work, family, and fitness commitments in your 40s. So not only will you be improving your physical health by doing cardio, but you'll also be boosting your mental well-being.

When it comes to weight loss, consistency is key. It's important to find a cardio routine that you enjoy and that fits into your busy schedule. Whether you prefer to hit the gym before work, go for a jog during your lunch break, or take a dance class in the evening, make sure to carve out time for your workouts each day. By staying consistent with your cardio routine, you'll not only see the pounds start to melt away, but you'll also improve your overall fitness level and energy levels.

Remember, it's never too late to start incorporating cardiovascular exercise into your routine. Whether you're new to working out or have been active for years, adding in regular cardio sessions can help you reach your weight loss goals and improve your overall health and well-being. So lace up your sneakers, grab your water bottle, and get moving – your body and mind will thank you for it!

Nutrition Tips for Building Muscle and Losing Weight

If you're over 40 and looking to build muscle and lose weight, it's important to focus on your nutrition. Eating a balanced diet that is rich in protein, healthy fats, and complex carbohydrates can help support your fitness goals. Make sure to include plenty of fruits, vegetables, and whole grains in your meals to provide your body with the nutrients it needs to fuel your workouts and recover properly.

To build muscle and lose weight effectively, it's essential to pay attention to your portion sizes and meal timing. Eating smaller, frequent meals throughout the day can help keep your metabolism revved up and prevent overeating. Aim to include a source of protein in each meal and snack to support muscle growth and repair. Don't forget to stay hydrated by drinking plenty of water throughout the day to keep your energy levels up and aid in digestion.

In addition to focusing on your diet, incorporating strength training and cardiovascular exercise into your fitness routine can help you achieve your muscle-building and weight loss goals. Strength training exercises like weightlifting and bodyweight exercises can help increase muscle mass and boost your metabolism. Cardiovascular exercises like running, cycling, or swimming can help burn calories and improve your cardiovascular health.

It's important to listen to your body and give yourself rest days to allow for proper recovery. Overtraining can lead to burnout and increase your risk of injury, so make sure to schedule in rest days and prioritize sleep to support your body's recovery process. Don't forget to incorporate flexibility and mobility exercises into your routine to improve your range of motion and prevent injuries.

Remember, building muscle and losing weight takes time and consistency. Stay motivated by setting realistic goals and tracking your progress along the way. Celebrate your achievements, no matter how small, and don't be too hard on yourself if you have setbacks. By staying consistent with your nutrition, exercise, and recovery, you can achieve your fitness goals and maintain a healthy lifestyle in your 40s.

Chapter 4: Improving Flexibility and Mobility

Importance of Stretching in Your 40s

Stretching is often an overlooked aspect of fitness, but it is crucial, especially as we age. In your 40s, your body may not be as limber as it once was, making it even more important to incorporate stretching into your routine. Stretching helps improve flexibility and mobility, which can help prevent injuries and improve your overall quality of life. By taking just a few minutes each day to stretch, you can keep your muscles and joints healthy and functioning properly.

As we get older, our muscles tend to lose elasticity and become tighter, which can lead to decreased range of motion and increased risk of injury. Stretching regularly can help counteract these effects, keeping your muscles supple and your joints mobile. This can be especially beneficial for those over 40 who may be experiencing age-related stiffness or joint pain. By incorporating stretching into your daily routine, you can maintain or even improve your flexibility and mobility, allowing you to stay active and engaged in the activities you love.

In addition to preventing injuries, stretching can also help improve your posture and balance, which can become increasingly important as we age. Poor posture can lead to aches and pains, as well as increased risk of falls. By stretching regularly, you can help correct muscle imbalances and improve your overall alignment, leading to better posture and balance. This can not only help prevent injuries, but also boost your confidence and overall sense of well-being.

Incorporating stretching into your fitness routine can also help you achieve your weight loss and muscle-building goals. By improving your flexibility and mobility, you can perform exercises with proper form, allowing you to target specific muscle groups more effectively. This can help you build lean muscle mass and increase your metabolism, making it easier to lose weight and maintain a healthy body composition. Additionally, stretching can help prevent muscle imbalances and reduce the risk of overuse injuries, allowing you to stay consistent with your fitness routine and reach your goals faster.

Overall, stretching is a crucial component of a balanced fitness routine, especially for those over 40. By taking the time to stretch regularly, you can improve your flexibility, mobility, posture, and balance, while also reducing your risk of injury and enhancing your performance in other areas of fitness. So, whether you're looking to lose weight, build muscle, or simply stay active and healthy in your 40s, don't forget to make stretching a priority in your daily routine. Your body will thank you for it!

Yoga and Pilates for Flexibility

In your 40s, maintaining flexibility becomes increasingly important for overall health and well-being. Incorporating yoga and Pilates into your fitness routine can help improve flexibility, mobility, and balance. These low-impact exercises focus on stretching and strengthening muscles, leading to increased flexibility and reduced risk of injury as you age.

Yoga, with its focus on breathing and mindfulness, not only improves flexibility but also promotes relaxation and reduces stress. By practicing yoga regularly, you can increase your range of motion, improve posture, and alleviate tension in your muscles and joints. Whether you're a beginner or an experienced yogi, there are classes and poses tailored to suit your needs and abilities.

Pilates, on the other hand, targets core strength and stability, which are essential for maintaining good posture and preventing back pain. By engaging in Pilates exercises that emphasize controlled movements and proper alignment, you can strengthen your muscles and improve flexibility without putting undue stress on your joints. These exercises can be modified to suit your fitness level, making them accessible to anyone over 40 looking to improve their flexibility.

Combining yoga and Pilates in your fitness routine can provide a well-rounded approach to improving flexibility and mobility in your 40s. Whether you choose to attend classes at a studio or practice at home, consistency is key to seeing results. Set aside time each week to dedicate to these exercises, and you'll soon notice improvements in your flexibility, balance, and overall well-being.

Remember, it's never too late to start prioritizing your flexibility and mobility. By incorporating yoga and Pilates into your fitness routine, you can enhance your physical and mental well-being, reduce the risk of age-related injuries, and feel more confident and capable in your everyday activities. Embrace the challenge, stay consistent, and enjoy the benefits of increased flexibility in your 40s and beyond.

Mobility Exercises for Joint Health

Mobility is key to maintaining joint health as we age, especially for those of us in our 40s. As we juggle work, family, and fitness commitments, it can be easy to neglect our bodies and forget the importance of

Chapter 5: Maintaining a Healthy Diet and Nutrition Plan

Balancing Macros for Optimal Health

When it comes to achieving optimal health in your 40s, one key component to focus on is balancing your macros. Macros, short for macronutrients, are the three main nutrients that make up our diet: carbohydrates, proteins, and fats. By paying attention to the balance of these macros in your daily meals, you can fuel your body properly, support weight loss and muscle building, and maintain overall health and well-being.

To achieve a balanced macro ratio, start by including a variety of whole foods in your diet. Aim to fill your plate with lean proteins such as chicken, fish, tofu, and legumes, complex carbohydrates like whole grains, fruits, and vegetables, and healthy fats from sources like avocados, nuts, and olive oil. By including all three macronutrients in each meal, you can ensure that your body is getting the nutrients it needs to function at its best.

In addition to balancing your macros, it's important to pay attention to portion sizes. As we age, our metabolism naturally slows down, making it easier to gain weight if we consume more calories than we burn. By practicing mindful eating and paying attention to portion sizes, you can prevent overeating and maintain a healthy weight. Consider using measuring cups or a food scale to help you accurately portion out your meals and snacks.

Another important aspect of balancing macros for optimal health is staying hydrated. Water is essential for digestion, nutrient absorption, and overall health. Aim to drink at least eight glasses of water per day, and consider adding in herbal teas or infused water for added flavor and hydration. Staying properly hydrated can also help curb cravings and prevent overeating, making it easier to stick to your healthy eating plan.

In conclusion, balancing macros for optimal health is a key component of maintaining a healthy diet and nutrition plan in your 40s. By including a variety of whole foods, paying attention to portion sizes, and staying hydrated, you can support weight loss, muscle building, and overall well-being. Remember, it's never too late to make positive changes to your diet and lifestyle. Start today by focusing on balancing your macros and fueling your body with the nutrients it needs to thrive.

Superfoods for Energy and Vitality

Are you struggling to keep up with the demands of life in your 40s? Do you find yourself feeling tired and drained more often than not? It's time to introduce some superfoods into your diet to boost your energy levels and vitality. These powerhouse foods are packed with nutrients that can help you stay active, alert, and ready to take on whatever life throws your way.

One of the best superfoods for energy and vitality is spinach. This leafy green is rich in iron, which helps oxygenate your blood and keep your energy levels up. It's also packed with vitamins and minerals that support overall health and well-being. Try adding spinach to your salads, smoothies, or stir-fries for a delicious and nutrient-packed boost.

Another superfood to consider is quinoa. This ancient grain is not only a great source of protein and fiber but also contains a good amount of iron and magnesium. These nutrients are essential for energy production and muscle function, making quinoa a great choice for anyone looking to stay active and energized.

Berries are also a fantastic superfood for energy and vitality. Blueberries, strawberries, and raspberries are all packed with antioxidants that can help fight inflammation and oxidative stress in the body. They're also low in calories and high in fiber, making them a great choice for anyone looking to maintain a healthy weight and boost their energy levels.

Incorporating these superfoods into your diet can make a big difference in how you feel and function on a daily basis. By fueling your body with nutrient-dense foods, you'll have the energy and vitality to tackle your work, family, and fitness commitments with ease. So go ahead and give these superfoods a try – your 40s will thank you for it!

Meal Prepping for Busy Schedules

Meal prepping is a game-changer when it comes to maintaining a healthy diet and nutrition plan, especially for those with busy schedules. As we navigate the challenges of work, family, and fitness commitments in our 40s, it can be easy to let our nutrition slip. However, by taking the time to plan and prepare meals in advance, we can ensure that we are fueling our bodies with the nutrients they need to thrive.

One of the key benefits of meal prepping is that it can help us overcome age-related fitness challenges. As we get older, our metabolism tends to slow down, making it harder to lose weight and build muscle. By preparing healthy, balanced meals ahead of time, we can ensure that we are getting the right mix of nutrients to support our fitness goals. Additionally, meal prepping can help us prevent and manage injuries by ensuring that we are eating foods that support our joint health and overall well-being.

Improving flexibility and mobility is another important aspect of staying active and healthy in our 40s. Meal prepping can help us achieve this goal by ensuring that we are eating foods rich in vitamins and minerals that support joint health and flexibility. By including a variety of fruits, vegetables, lean proteins, and whole grains in our meal prep plans, we can fuel our bodies with the nutrients they need to stay limber and agile.

Setting and achieving fitness goals can be a daunting task, especially with the demands of work and family life. However, meal prepping can help us stay on track by providing us with the fuel we need to power through our workouts and recover properly. By taking the time to plan and prepare our meals in advance, we can ensure that we are eating foods that support our fitness goals and help us stay motivated and consistent with our routine.

In conclusion, meal prepping is a valuable tool for anyone over 40 looking to balance work, family, and fitness commitments. By taking the time to plan and prepare meals in advance, we can ensure that we are fueling our bodies with the nutrients they need to thrive. Whether your goal is to lose weight, build muscle, improve flexibility, or boost your metabolism, meal prepping can help you achieve success in all areas of your fitness journey. So take the time to invest in your health and well-being by incorporating meal prepping into your routine – your body will thank you for it!

Chapter 6: Preventing and Managing Injuries

Listening to Your Body

Listening to your body is crucial as you navigate your fitness journey in your 40s. Our bodies are constantly sending us signals, letting us know what they need and how they are feeling. By tuning into these messages, you can better understand how to care for yourself and achieve your health and fitness goals. Whether it's aches and pains, fatigue, or cravings, your body is always speaking to you - it's up to you to listen.

As we age, our bodies may have different needs and limitations than they did in our younger years. By paying attention to how your body responds to different exercises, foods, and lifestyle choices, you can make adjustments to ensure you are supporting your overall health and well-being. This might mean incorporating more rest days into your workout routine, trying new forms of exercise to improve flexibility and mobility, or adjusting your diet to better fuel your body.

When it comes to losing weight and building muscle after 40, listening to your body is key. Pay attention to how certain foods make you feel, how your body responds to different types of exercise, and when you may need to dial back intensity to prevent injury. By being in tune with your body's signals, you can create a sustainable and effective fitness plan that works for you.

Improving flexibility and mobility in your 40s can help prevent injuries, improve posture, and enhance overall quality of life. By listening to your body and incorporating stretching, yoga, and mobility exercises into your routine, you can increase your range of motion and feel more comfortable in your daily activities. Remember, it's never too late to work on your flexibility and mobility - your body will thank you for it.

Incorporating regular check-ins with your body can help you stay on track with your fitness goals, boost your metabolism and energy levels, and prevent and manage injuries. By paying attention to how you feel before, during, and after workouts, meals, and daily activities, you can make informed choices that support your health and well-being. Remember, your body is your most valuable asset - listen to it, respect it, and take care of it.

Proper Warm-Up and Cool Down Techniques

Proper Warm-Up and Cool Down Techniques are crucial for anyone over 40 looking to maintain a healthy and active lifestyle. As we age, our bodies require a little extra care and attention to prevent injuries and stay in top shape. By incorporating these techniques into your fitness routine, you can improve your overall performance, flexibility, and mobility, while reducing the risk of strains and sprains.

Before starting any workout, it's important to warm up your muscles and prepare your body for the physical activity ahead. A proper warm-up should include dynamic stretches, light cardio, and mobility exercises to increase blood flow and flexibility. This will help loosen up tight muscles and joints, reducing the risk of injury during your workout. Take the time to gently ease into your routine, allowing your body to adjust and warm up gradually.

After completing your workout, don't forget to cool down and stretch your muscles to prevent stiffness and soreness. Cool down exercises help lower your heart rate and promote muscle recovery, aiding in the prevention of muscle fatigue and injury. Incorporate static stretches and foam rolling into your post-workout routine to help maintain flexibility and improve muscle recovery. This will also help reduce the buildup of lactic acid in your muscles, reducing soreness and promoting faster recovery.

By incorporating proper warm-up and cool down techniques into your fitness routine, you can improve your overall performance and reduce the risk of injuries. Remember to listen to your body and adjust your routine as needed to prevent overexertion and strain. With consistency and dedication, you can achieve your fitness goals and maintain a healthy and active lifestyle well into your 40s and beyond.

Don't let age be a barrier to achieving your fitness goals. By incorporating proper warm-up and cool down techniques into your routine, you can stay motivated and consistent with your workouts, prevent injuries, and improve your overall fitness and mobility. Take the time to care for your body and prioritize your health and well-being. With the right approach and mindset, you can overcome age-related fitness challenges and achieve success in your fitness journey.

Seeking Professional Help When Needed

Seeking professional help when needed is a crucial step in achieving your fitness goals in your 40s. As we age, our bodies may require more specialized care and attention to ensure we are staying healthy and active. Whether you are looking to lose weight, build muscle, improve flexibility, or simply maintain a healthy lifestyle, seeking guidance from a professional can make a world of difference in your journey.

It's important to remember that age-related fitness challenges are common, but they are not insurmountable. By working with a fitness trainer, physical therapist, or nutritionist, you can tailor a plan that is specifically designed to meet your needs and goals. These professionals have the expertise to help you navigate any obstacles you may encounter and provide you with the tools and support you need to succeed.

Maintaining a healthy diet and nutrition plan is essential for overall health and well-being, especially as we age. A nutritionist can help you create a balanced meal plan that supports your fitness goals and provides you with the energy you need to stay active and engaged in your daily life. They can also help you navigate any dietary restrictions or health issues you may have, ensuring that you are getting the nutrients your body needs to thrive.

In addition to physical health, it's important to prioritize your mental and emotional well-being as well. Seeking support from a therapist or counselor can help you manage stress, anxiety, or any other mental health challenges that may be impacting your ability to stay motivated and consistent with your fitness routine. Taking care of your mental health is just as important as taking care of your physical health, and seeking professional help when needed is a powerful step in achieving balance in all areas of your life.

Remember, it's never too late to seek professional help and make positive changes in your life. By working with a team of experts who can support you on your fitness journey, you can overcome any obstacles you may face and achieve your goals with confidence and determination. Don't be afraid to ask for help - you deserve to live a healthy, active, and fulfilling life in your 40s and beyond.

Chapter 7: Boosting Metabolism and Energy Levels

Incorporating HIIT Workouts

Incorporating HIIT workouts into your fitness routine can be a game-changer, especially for those of us in our 40s. High Intensity Interval Training (HIIT) is a form of exercise that involves short bursts of intense activity followed by brief rest periods. Not only does HIIT help you burn more calories in less time, but it also boosts your metabolism, increases muscle mass, and improves cardiovascular health. It's a great way to lose weight and build muscle after 40, all while keeping your workouts efficient and effective.

One of the key benefits of HIIT workouts is their ability to improve flexibility and mobility in your 40s. As we age, our muscles and joints can become stiff and less flexible, making it harder to move freely and perform everyday tasks. Incorporating HIIT exercises that focus on full-body movements can help increase your range of motion, improve joint flexibility, and enhance overall mobility. This can not only prevent injuries but also make daily activities easier and more enjoyable.

Maintaining a healthy diet and nutrition plan is essential for achieving optimal results with HIIT workouts. Eating a balanced diet rich in lean proteins, whole grains, fruits, and vegetables can provide your body with the fuel it needs to perform at its best during high-intensity exercise. It's important to fuel your body before and after your workouts to support muscle recovery, energy levels, and overall health. By combining HIIT workouts with a nutritious diet, you can maximize your results and feel your best in your 40s.

Overcoming age-related fitness challenges can be tough, but HIIT workouts offer a solution that is both effective and efficient. By incorporating HIIT into your routine, you can boost your metabolism and energy levels, making it easier to stay active and motivated. HIIT workouts can be modified to fit your fitness level and preferences, allowing you to progress at your own pace while still challenging yourself. This flexibility makes HIIT a great option for anyone looking to prevent and manage injuries while staying active in their 40s.

Setting and achieving fitness goals in your 40s can be challenging, but with the right mindset and tools, it is definitely possible. HIIT workouts can help you stay motivated and consistent with your fitness routine by providing variety, intensity, and results. By balancing work, family, and fitness commitments, you can create a sustainable and fulfilling lifestyle that supports your health and well-being. Incorporating HIIT into your routine can help you achieve your fitness goals, overcome age-related challenges, and feel your best in your 40s and beyond.

Hydrating Properly for Energy

Hydrating properly is crucial for maintaining energy levels, especially as we age. As we hit our 40s, our bodies may not be as efficient at retaining water, leading to dehydration and fatigue. To combat this, it's important to make a conscious effort to drink enough water throughout the day. Aim for at least 8-10 glasses of water daily, and even more if you are engaging in vigorous exercise or spending time outdoors in hot weather. By staying hydrated, you can boost your metabolism and energy levels, helping you feel more alert and focused throughout the day.

In addition to drinking water, consider incorporating other hydrating beverages into your routine, such as herbal teas, coconut water, or infused water with fruits and herbs. These options can add flavor and variety to your hydration plan while still providing the necessary fluids your body needs to function optimally. Remember, caffeinated and alcoholic beverages can have a diuretic effect, so it's best to consume them in moderation and balance them out with plenty of water.

When it comes to staying hydrated, timing is key. Start your day with a glass of water to kickstart your metabolism and rehydrate after a night's sleep. Throughout the day, drink water before, during, and after meals to aid in digestion and absorption of nutrients. Keep a water bottle with you at all times as a reminder to stay hydrated, and consider setting alarms or reminders on your phone to prompt you to drink water regularly.

Proper hydration is not only important for maintaining energy levels but also for preventing injuries and managing age-related fitness challenges. Dehydration can lead to muscle cramps, fatigue, and decreased performance during workouts, putting you at risk for accidents or overexertion. By prioritizing hydration and making it a consistent part of your daily routine, you can stay active, healthy, and injury-free well into your 40s and beyond.

Remember, staying hydrated is a simple yet powerful way to support your overall health and well-being. By making a conscious effort to drink enough water and other hydrating beverages, you can boost your energy levels, improve your metabolism, and enhance your performance in both your workouts and daily activities. So, grab that water bottle, take a sip, and feel the difference that proper hydration can make in your life.

Getting Sufficient Sleep for Recovery

Getting sufficient sleep is crucial for recovery, especially as we age. As we hit our 40s, our bodies require more rest to repair and rejuvenate from the daily stresses we put them through. Lack of sleep can lead to increased cortisol levels, decreased muscle recovery, and overall decreased performance in our fitness goals. By prioritizing sleep and aiming for 7-9 hours each night, we can optimize our body's ability to recover and thrive.

When it comes to losing weight and building muscle after 40, sleep plays a significant role. During deep sleep stages, our bodies release growth hormones that aid in muscle repair and growth. Additionally, proper rest helps regulate hunger hormones, preventing overeating and aiding in weight loss. By making sleep a priority, we can support our weight loss and muscle-building efforts, leading to better overall fitness results.

Improving flexibility and mobility in your 40s can also benefit from adequate sleep. Rest allows our muscles to relax and lengthen, reducing stiffness and improving range of motion. This can help prevent injuries and enhance performance in activities such as yoga, pilates, or weightlifting. By getting enough sleep, we can support our body's ability to move freely and maintain flexibility as we age.

Maintaining a healthy diet and nutrition plan in your 40s is essential for overall wellness, but did you know that sleep can impact our food choices? Lack of sleep can lead to increased cravings for sugary and high-fat foods, making it harder to stick to a healthy eating plan. By getting enough rest, we can regulate our hunger hormones and make better food choices, supporting our fitness goals and overall health. Remember, sleep is a key component of a balanced approach to nutrition and fitness in your 40s.

In conclusion, prioritizing sleep is a crucial aspect of maintaining a healthy and active lifestyle in your 40s. By getting enough rest, we can support our weight loss and muscle-building efforts, improve flexibility and mobility, maintain a healthy diet, prevent injuries, boost our metabolism and energy levels, and stay motivated and consistent with our fitness routine. Remember, sleep is not a luxury but a necessity for optimal health and wellness, so make it a priority in your daily routine. Your body will thank you for it!

Chapter 8: Setting and Achieving Fitness Goals

SMART Goal Setting

Setting SMART goals is essential for anyone over 40 who wants to achieve their fitness and health objectives. SMART stands for Specific, Measurable, Achievable, Relevant, and Time-bound. By following this framework, you can create a roadmap to success that will keep you motivated and on track towards your desired outcomes.

When setting fitness goals in your 40s, it's important to be specific about what you want to achieve. Instead of saying you want to "lose weight," try setting a goal like "I want to lose 10 pounds in three months by exercising three times a week and eating a balanced diet." This specificity will give you a clear target to work towards and help you stay focused on your ultimate goal.

In addition to being specific, your goals should also be measurable. This means setting concrete metrics to track your progress. For example, if your goal is to improve flexibility and mobility, you could measure your progress by tracking how far you can reach during a stretch or how long it takes you to complete a certain yoga pose. By measuring your progress, you can celebrate small victories along the way and stay motivated to keep pushing forward.

Another key component of SMART goal setting is ensuring your goals are achievable. It's important to set goals that challenge you but are also within reach. For example, if you've never run a marathon before, setting a goal to complete one in six months may not be realistic. Instead, start with a smaller goal like running a 5k and gradually work your way up to longer distances. By setting achievable goals, you'll build confidence in your abilities and set yourself up for success.

Lastly, your goals should be time-bound, meaning you set a deadline for when you want to achieve them. By giving yourself a timeframe to work towards, you create a sense of urgency and hold yourself accountable for making progress. Whether your goal is to lose weight, build muscle, or improve your overall fitness, setting a deadline will keep you focused and motivated to stay on track. Remember, age is just a number, and with the right mindset and SMART goal-setting strategies, you can achieve your fitness goals and lead a healthier, more active lifestyle in your 40s and beyond.

Tracking Progress and Adjusting Goals

Tracking progress and adjusting goals are crucial aspects of maintaining a healthy and active lifestyle in your 40s. As we age, our bodies require different types of exercise and nutrition to stay strong and fit. By keeping track of your progress, you can identify areas where you may need to make adjustments to reach your fitness goals. Whether you are looking to lose weight, build muscle, improve flexibility, or boost your metabolism, tracking your progress is key to success.

One of the best ways to track your progress is by keeping a fitness journal. Write down your workouts, meals, and how you are feeling both physically and mentally. This will allow you to see patterns and make adjustments as needed. If you notice that you are not making progress in a certain area, it may be time to reassess your goals and make changes to your routine. Remember, progress is not always linear, and it is important to celebrate small victories along the way.

In addition to tracking your progress, it is important to regularly reassess your fitness goals. As we age, our bodies may respond differently to exercise and nutrition, so it is important to adjust your goals accordingly. If you find that a certain goal is no longer realistic or achievable, don't be afraid to change it. Setting realistic and achievable goals is key to staying motivated and consistent with your fitness routine.

When adjusting your goals, it is important to be kind to yourself. It is easy to get discouraged when progress is slow or setbacks occur, but remember that fitness is a journey, not a destination. Be patient with yourself and trust the process. Surround yourself with positive influences and seek support from friends, family, or a fitness coach if needed. Remember, you are capable of achieving your fitness goals, no matter your age.

By tracking your progress and adjusting your goals as needed, you can stay on track towards a healthier and more active lifestyle in your 40s. Remember to celebrate your achievements, no matter how small, and stay motivated to continue working towards your goals. With dedication, consistency, and a positive mindset, you can overcome age-related fitness challenges and achieve the best version of yourself.

Celebrating Achievements Along the Way

As we journey through our 40s, it's important to take a moment to pause and celebrate the achievements we've made along the way. Whether it's losing a few pounds, improving our flexibility, or simply staying consistent with our fitness routine, every small victory is worth celebrating. These milestones not only show our progress but also serve as motivation to keep pushing forward towards our goals.

In the realm of fitness, it's common to set lofty goals and strive for perfection. However, it's essential to remember that progress is not always linear. There will be ups and downs, setbacks and breakthroughs. By taking the time to acknowledge and celebrate the small wins, we can stay motivated and focused on the bigger picture. So, whether you've finally mastered that yoga pose or increased your weightlifting capacity, be sure to give yourself a pat on the back for a job well done.

When it comes to maintaining a healthy diet and nutrition plan in your 40s, consistency is key. It's easy to get caught up in the latest fad diets or extreme workout regimens, but the real success lies in finding a sustainable approach that works for you. By celebrating the small victories, such as choosing a nutritious meal over fast food or resisting the urge to indulge in sugary snacks, you are reinforcing positive habits that will benefit you in the long run.

Overcoming age-related fitness challenges can be daunting, but it's important to remember that progress is possible at any age. By focusing on small achievements, such as improving your mobility or increasing your endurance, you can build confidence and momentum towards your larger goals. Celebrate these victories as a testament to your resilience and determination to defy the limitations often associated with aging.

In the balancing act of work, family, and fitness commitments, it's easy to feel overwhelmed and discouraged. However, by taking a moment to acknowledge and celebrate your achievements, you can find the motivation to keep going. Remember, every step forward, no matter how small, is a step in the right direction. So, celebrate your wins, no matter how big or small, and keep pushing towards a healthier, happier you in your 40s and beyond.

Chapter 9: Staying Motivated and Consistent

Finding Your Why

In the journey to living a healthy and fulfilling life in your 40s, one of the most important things to consider is finding your "why." This means understanding the reasons behind your desire to improve your health and fitness, and using those motivations to fuel your actions. Whether it's wanting to lose weight, build muscle, improve flexibility, or boost your energy levels, having a clear and powerful reason for why you want to make these changes can make all the difference in your success.

When you take the time to truly reflect on your "why," you may uncover deep-seated desires to live a longer, happier life, to set a positive example for your children, or to simply feel more confident and comfortable in your own skin. Whatever your reasons may be, knowing them and connecting with them on a personal level can give you the strength and determination to push through any obstacles that may come your way.

It's not always easy to stay motivated and consistent with your fitness routine, especially when balancing work, family, and other commitments. But by anchoring yourself in your "why," you can remind yourself of the bigger picture and stay focused on your goals. When you hit a rough patch or feel like giving up, take a moment to revisit your motivations and remember why you started this journey in the first place.

In addition to helping you stay on track with your fitness goals, finding your "why" can also help you overcome age-related challenges that may arise. As we get older, our bodies may not respond to exercise and diet changes as quickly as they once did. But by understanding your motivations and staying committed to your health and well-being, you can navigate these obstacles with grace and determination.

So take some time to dig deep and discover your "why." Whether it's wanting to feel stronger, look better, or simply live a more fulfilling life, knowing your reasons for wanting to improve your health and fitness can be the driving force that propels you towards success in your 40s and beyond. Remember, your "why" is your North Star – let it guide you on your journey to a healthier, happier you.

Creating a Supportive Environment

Creating a supportive environment is crucial when it comes to achieving your fitness goals in your 40s. As we age, it becomes even more important to surround ourselves with positivity and encouragement to stay motivated and consistent with our fitness routines. Whether you are looking to lose weight, build muscle, improve flexibility, or boost your metabolism, having a supportive environment can make all the difference in your success.

One way to create a supportive environment is to surround yourself with like-minded individuals who share similar fitness goals. Joining a fitness group or finding a workout buddy can provide you with the accountability and motivation you need to stay on track. Having someone to cheer you on and celebrate your progress can make all the difference in staying committed to your fitness journey.

Another way to create a supportive environment is to make your home a place that fosters healthy habits. Stocking your kitchen with nutritious foods and meal prepping can make it easier to stick to a healthy diet and nutrition plan. Creating a designated workout space in your home can also make it more convenient to squeeze in a workout, even on busy days. By setting up your environment for success, you are more likely to stay on track with your fitness goals.

In addition to setting up your physical environment for success, it is important to also focus on your mental and emotional well-being. Surround yourself with positive affirmations, inspirational quotes, and reminders of why you started your fitness journey in the first place. Taking care of your mental health and finding ways to manage stress can help you stay motivated and consistent with your fitness routine, even when life gets busy.

Overall, creating a supportive environment is essential for anyone over 40 looking to achieve their fitness goals. By surrounding yourself with positive influences, setting up your physical environment for success, and focusing on your mental and emotional well-being, you can overcome age-related fitness challenges and stay on track with your health and wellness goals. Remember, you deserve to prioritize your well-being and create a space that supports your journey to a healthier, happier you.

Rewarding Yourself for Consistency

Congratulations on making it this far in your fitness journey! Consistency is key when it comes to reaching your health and wellness goals, especially as we age. It's important to acknowledge and reward yourself for the hard work and dedication you've put into maintaining a healthy lifestyle in your 40s. By staying consistent with your fitness routine, you are setting yourself up for long-term success and improved overall well-being.

One way to reward yourself for consistency is to celebrate your progress, no matter how small. Whether you've lost a few pounds, increased your flexibility, or hit a new personal best in the gym, take the time to acknowledge and celebrate these achievements. Treat yourself to a massage, a new workout outfit, or a healthy meal at your favorite restaurant. These small rewards can help keep you motivated and on track to reaching your fitness goals.

Another way to reward yourself for consistency is to prioritize self-care and relaxation. As we age, it's important to listen to our bodies and give them the rest and recovery they need. Treat yourself to a spa day, a leisurely walk in nature, or a relaxing yoga class. Taking care of your mental and emotional well-being is just as important as taking care of your physical health.

In addition to celebrating your progress and prioritizing self-care, consider setting new fitness goals to challenge yourself and keep things interesting. By constantly striving to improve and push yourself out of your comfort zone, you can continue to see progress and growth in your fitness journey. Whether it's running a 5k, mastering a new yoga pose, or increasing your weightlifting capacity, setting and achieving new goals can help keep you motivated and consistent.

Remember, consistency is not about perfection. It's about showing up for yourself day in and day out, even when life gets busy or obstacles arise. By rewarding yourself for your consistency and dedication to your health and fitness, you are investing in your future self and setting a positive example for those around you. Keep up the great work, and don't forget to celebrate your wins along the way!

Chapter 10: Balancing Work, Family, and Fitness Commitments

Time Management Strategies

Time management is essential when it comes to achieving your fitness goals in your 40s. With a busy schedule juggling work, family, and other commitments, finding the time to exercise and prioritize your health can be challenging. However, by implementing effective time management strategies, you can make fitness a priority in your daily routine.

One key strategy for better time management is to schedule your workouts in advance. By blocking out specific times in your calendar for exercise, you are more likely to stick to your routine and avoid skipping workouts. Whether it's early in the morning before work, during your lunch break, or in the evening after dinner, find a time that works best for you and commit to it.

Another helpful time management tip is to prioritize high-intensity, efficient workouts that maximize your time and results. Instead of spending hours at the gym, focus on short, intense workouts that target multiple muscle groups and elevate your heart rate. This way, you can get an effective workout in less time, allowing you to fit fitness into even the busiest of schedules.

In addition to scheduling your workouts and focusing on efficiency, it's important to incorporate movement throughout your day. Look for opportunities to be active, whether it's taking the stairs instead of the elevator, going for a walk during your lunch break, or doing bodyweight exercises while watching TV. By staying active throughout the day, you can boost your metabolism, increase energy levels, and improve overall fitness.

By implementing these time management strategies, you can overcome age-related fitness challenges, stay motivated and consistent with your fitness routine, and achieve your health and wellness goals in your 40s. Remember, prioritizing your health is not selfish – it's essential for maintaining a strong body, sharp mind, and fulfilling life. With proper time management, you can balance work, family, and fitness commitments while feeling your best at any age.

Incorporating Family into Fitness Activities

Incorporating family into fitness activities can be a fun and rewarding way to stay active and healthy in your 40s. Not only does it provide an opportunity to bond with your loved ones, but it also sets a positive example for your children or grandchildren. By involving your family in your fitness routine, you can instill healthy habits that will benefit them for years to come.

One way to incorporate family into fitness activities is to plan active outings together. Whether it's going for a family hike, bike ride, or swim, there are plenty of ways to get moving as a group. Not only does this promote physical activity, but it also creates lasting memories that you can cherish together.

Another way to involve your family in fitness activities is to turn household chores into a workout. Instead of dreading cleaning the house or working in the yard, turn it into a family fitness challenge. Set a timer and see who can clean the fastest or do the most squats while gardening. Not only does this make chores more enjoyable, but it also helps you stay active throughout the day.

Meal planning and cooking can also be a great way to involve your family in your fitness journey. Get your kids or partner involved in choosing healthy recipes, grocery shopping, and preparing meals together. Not only does this teach valuable cooking skills, but it also ensures that everyone is eating nutritious meals that support your fitness goals.

Overall, incorporating family into fitness activities is a great way to stay motivated and consistent with your routine. By involving your loved ones in your fitness journey, you can create a supportive environment that encourages everyone to prioritize their health and well-being. So why not make fitness a family affair and enjoy the benefits of staying active together in your 40s and beyond.

Prioritizing Self-Care for Overall Well-Being

Prioritizing self-care is crucial for overall well-being, especially as we navigate our 40s and beyond. It's easy to get caught up in the demands of work, family, and other commitments, but taking care of yourself should always be a top priority. By focusing on self-care, you can improve your physical health, mental well-being, and overall quality of life.

One key aspect of self-care in your 40s is maintaining a healthy diet and nutrition plan. As we age, our bodies may require different nutrients and dietary guidelines to support optimal health. By eating a balanced diet rich in fruits, vegetables, lean proteins, and whole grains, you can fuel your body and mind for peak performance. Don't forget to stay hydrated and listen to your body's hunger cues to ensure you're meeting your nutritional needs.

In addition to eating well, it's important to stay active and prioritize fitness in your 40s. Regular exercise can help you lose weight, build muscle, improve flexibility and mobility, boost your metabolism, and increase energy levels. Whether you prefer strength training, cardio, yoga, or another form of exercise, finding activities that you enjoy and that fit your lifestyle is key to staying consistent and motivated.

While staying active is important, it's also crucial to prevent and manage injuries as you age. Pay attention to any aches or pains, and don't push yourself too hard if you're feeling fatigued or sore. Incorporating rest days, proper warm-ups and cool-downs, and listening to your body's signals can help you stay injury-free and on track with your fitness goals.

Lastly, don't forget to make time for self-care activities that nurture your mental and emotional well-being. Whether it's meditation, journaling, spending time with loved ones, or pursuing hobbies and interests, taking care of your mental health is just as important as taking care of your physical health. By prioritizing self-care in all aspects of your life, you can achieve balance, fulfillment, and overall well-being in your 40s and beyond.

Conclusion: Embracing the Balancing Act in Your 40s

In conclusion, embracing the balancing act in your 40s is crucial for maintaining a healthy and fulfilling lifestyle. As we age, it becomes even more important to prioritize our physical and mental well-being. By finding the right balance between work, family, and fitness commitments, you can achieve optimal health and happiness in this stage of life.

One key aspect of this balancing act is staying active and fit. It's never too late to start or continue a fitness routine that works for you. Whether it's strength training, yoga, or cardio, finding activities that you enjoy and that challenge you is essential for maintaining muscle mass, flexibility, and overall health in your 40s.

Another important factor to consider is your diet and nutrition plan. As we age, our metabolism tends to slow down, making it easier to gain weight. By focusing on whole, nutrient-rich foods and staying hydrated, you can support your body's needs and maintain a healthy weight. Remember, it's not about perfection, but progress. Small changes over time can lead to significant improvements in your overall health and well-being.

It's also essential to listen to your body and prevent injuries while staying active. Pay attention to any aches or pains and modify your workouts accordingly. Incorporating proper warm-ups, stretches, and cooldowns can help improve flexibility and mobility, reducing your risk of injury and allowing you to stay active for years to come.

Lastly, remember to set achievable fitness goals and stay motivated and consistent with your routine. Celebrate your successes, no matter how small, and don't be discouraged by setbacks. By staying committed to your health and wellness in your 40s, you can enjoy a vibrant and fulfilling life for years to come. Embrace the balancing act, and you'll reap the rewards of a healthy and balanced lifestyle.